# MEDICAL
# EMERGENCIES
## *in the Physician's*
## *Office*

# MEDICAL EMERGENCIES
## *in the Physician's Office*

**Shirley Laidley, AHI, N.A.E.M.T.I/C**
National Registry First Responder, CPR Instructor

PEARSON
Prentice Hall

Upper Saddle River, New Jersey 07458

Library of Congress Cataloging-in-Publication Data

Laidley, Shirley.
  Medical emergencies in the physician's office / Shirley Laidley.—1st ed.
    p. ; cm.
  Includes index.
  ISBN-13: 978-0-13-239165-8
  ISBN-10:   0-13-239165-1
  1. Medical emergencies—Handbooks, manuals, etc. 2. Medical offices—
Handbooks, manuals, etc. I. Title.
  [DNLM: 1. Emergency Treatment—methods—Handbooks.
2. Emergencies—Handbooks. 3. Emergency Medicine—methods—
Handbooks. 4. Physicians' Offices—Handbooks. WB 39 L185m 2008]
  RC86.7.L335  2008
  616.02'5—dc22                   2007024841

Pearson Education LTD.          Pearson Education Australia PTY, Limited
Pearson Education Singapore, Pte. Ltd  Pearson Education North Asia Ltd
Pearson Education, Canada, Ltd     Pearson Educacion de Mexico, S.A. de C.V.
Pearson Education—Japan        Pearson Education Malaysia, Pte. Ltd

10 9 8 7 6 5 4 3

ISBN-13: 978-0-13-239165-8
ISBN-10:  0-13-239165-1

For my husband, Timothy, for his support
and encouragement.

# CONTENTS

This handy pocket book is a quick reference tool for anyone who might have to provide emergency medical care. This includes everyone from those with basic first aid knowledge, to medical assistants, and even to those working in emergency rooms. The book discusses many types of emergency situations and outlines a plan for handling each emergence covered.

## ORGANIZATION

Time is critical in an emergency situation. Treatment at the onset of an emergency can save lives. The emergencies covered in this quick reference book are presented in alphabetic order to help the reader find pertinent information quickly.

Trauma is described in many forms. Sometimes the patient is unaware of what exactly happened. Alternatively, the patient is unconscious and unable to communicate with the responder. Another emergency can be medical onset, with the patient in a trauma crisis. Treatment depends on medical and trauma assessments. Ensuring scene safety and attending to life-threatening airway, breathing, circulation (ABCs) symptoms are the most important tasks of the responder.

## REFUSAL OF CARE

The patient has the right to refuse care but only as long as he or she is not in a critical or life-threatening situation. The health care provider should have the patient sign a release form. This form will release the health care provider from any obligations of treatment.

If the patient's condition worsens to a life-threatening state or the patient becomes unconscious, then the health care provider may assist with any medical treatment needed. Emergency care would be provided according to the implied consent rule.

## REVIEWER PANEL

The invaluable editorial advice and direction provided by the following educators is deeply appreciated:

Cindy A. Abel, BS, CMA, PBT(ASCP)
Medical Assisting Program Chair
Ivy Tech Community College
Lafayette, IN

Kendra J. Allen, LPN
Ohio Institute of Health Careers
Columbus, OH

Michaelann Marie Allen, M.Ed., CMA
Program Coordinator/Instructor Medical Assisting
  Program
North Seattle Community College
Seattle, WA

Jennifer Barr, MT, M.Ed., CMA
Chairperson, Medical Assistant Technology
Sinclair Community College
Dayton, OH

Suzanne Bitters, RMA-NCPT/NCICS
(Certified American Red Cross Instructor)

Former Instructor/Senior Phlebotomist-CPR/
    FA Instructor
CHI Institute
Southampton, PA

Lou M. Brown, MT(ASCP), CMA
Program Director
Wayne Community College
Goldsboro, NC

Mindy Brown, RMA
Medical Assisting Instructor
Pima Medical Institute
Colorado Springs, CO

Denise Carsillo, MS, BS, RMA, BXMO
Allied Health Education Supervisor
New England Tech
Palm Beach Gardens, FL

Lisa L. Cook, CMA
Education Chair
Bryman College
Orchard, WA

Susan DeGirolamo, RMA, MCPT, NCICS
(Certified American Red Cross Instructor)
Medical Program Director
CHI Institute
Southampton, PA

Litta Dennis, MS, BSN
Adjunct Faculty Health Careers

Miami Dade College
Miami, FL

Evie O'Nan, RMA, EMT-B
Director of Health Care Education
National College,
Florence, KY

Shelly Rainer, LPN, RMA
Medical Instructor/Extern Coordinator
Vatterott College
Springfield, MO

Deanna T. Rieke, MS, BSN
Program Director, Medical Assisting
MSU-Billings, College of Technology
Billings, MT

Gary Shandrew, MS
Campus Director
Certified Careers Institute
Clearfield, UT

Lynn Slack, CMA
Medical Programs Director
ICM School of Business & Medical Careers
Pittsburgh, PA

Donna Stevenson, BA, LPN
Allied Health Department Chair
Remington College,
Largo, FL

# 1. Abdominal Injuries

## SUBJECTIVE/OBJECTIVE

Use the **OPQRST** Method to determine the patient's level of pain and discomfort:
- Onset
- Provocation
- Quality
- Radiation
- Severity
- Time

Use **SAMPLE** to determine the patient's history:
- S—OPQRST
- Allergies
- Medications
- Pertinent history
- Last oral intake
- Events leading to the pain

## ABDOMINAL CONDITIONS

- Appendicitis
- Cholecystitis/gallstones
- Pancreatitis
- Ulcer/internal bleeding
- Abdominal aortic aneurysm
- Hernia
- Renal colic
- Crohn's disease
- Irritable bowel syndrome
- Hepatitis

- Hiatal hernia
- Constipation
- Diarrhea

## ASSESSMENT/PLAN

- Perform primary assessment:
  —Airway
  —Breathing
  —Circulation
- Check vital signs every 2 minutes.
- Take SAMPLE history.

## PENETRATING WOUNDS

Penetrating abdominal wounds are related to wounds in other areas of the body. An object can enter the abdominal cavity and move upward toward the diaphragm. Do not remove the object. Secure it to the body. Any wounds to the abdominal area should be classified as life threatening.

## SUBJECTIVE/OBJECTIVE

- Intolerable pain
- Nausea
- Weakness
- Thirst
- Lacerations or puncture wounds to the abdominal area
- Contusions—blunt trauma
- Shock
- Coughing up blood
- Distended abdominal area
- Bleeding from entrance and exit wounds
- Organs protruding through an open wound

## ASSESSMENT/PLAN

- Lay patient in supine position.
- Perform primary assessment:
  —Airway
  —Breathing
  —Circulation
- Protruding organs—Pour sterile saline solution on wound and cover with sterile gauze. Never try to push organs back into abdominal cavity.
- Treat for shock.
- Check vital signs every 2 minutes.
- Document all findings concerning the patient's condition.

# 2. Allergic Reaction/ Anaphylaxis/ Anaphylactic Shock

## CAUSES OF AN ALLERGIC REACTION

- Plants
- Medications
- Insects
- Environmental
- Foods
- Household

## SUBJECTIVE/OBJECTIVE

- Shortness of breath
- Itching
- Rash
- Nausea/vomiting

## ASSESSMENT/EVALUATION

- Skin
  —Itching
  —Hives
  —Flushing
  —Swelling
  —Warm to touch
  —Discoloration
  —Rash

- Respiratory
  —Tightness in the throat and chest
  —Cough
  —Rapid breathing
  —Labored breathing
  —Stridor
  —Wheezing
  —Swelling of the tongue
- Cardiac
  —Increased heart rate—tachycardia
  —Decreased blood pressure B/P
- Generalized findings
  —Itchy, watery eyes
  —Headache
  —Runny nose
- Shock
  —Level of consciousness
  —Flushed, dry skin
  —Nausea/vomiting
  —Changes in vital signs
  —Increased pulse
  —Increased respirations
  —Decreased blood pressure
  —Cyanotic

## PLAN

- Inform the physician of the subjective and objective symptoms of the patient.
- Perform primary assessment:
  —Airway
  —Breathing
  —Circulation
- Treat for Choking.

- Allow the person to assume the position of greatest comfort—usually leaning forward, legs dangling.
- Monitor vital signs—pulse and BP—every 2 minutes.
- Treat for signs of shock.
- Assist conscious patients with the epinephrine autoinjector pen.
- Assist patients in taking medications as per physician's order.
- Document all findings and treatment concerning the allergic reaction.

# 3. *Altered Mental Status*

The functioning of the mind—normal or abnormal for that individual

## SUBJECTIVE/OBJECTIVE

- Fever and Headache—onset, duration and progression of symptoms
- Seizures
- Trauma/medical emergencies
- Medical or psychiatric history
- Any evidence of medication or drug use or exposure to toxins in the environment

## ASSESSMENT/EVALUATION

Check for the following:
- Vital signs
- Level of consciousness
- Any signs of trauma
- Odor of breath
- Any evidence of drug abuse
- Any medical alert tags
- Blood glucose level

## PLAN

- Inform the physician of the subjective and objective symptoms of the patient.
- Perform primary assessment:
  —Airway
  —Breathing
  —Circulation

- Be aware of a change in the patient's behavior.
  —Call police if behavior turns hostile.
- Check vital signs every 2 minutes.
- Give glucose if the patient's sugar levels are low.
- Assist the patient in taking medications as per physician's order.
- Document all findings and treatment concerning the behavior of the patient.

Altered Mental Status

# 4. Assessment—Conscious Patient

- Ask the patient:
  —What happened?
  —Where does it hurt?
  —Can you move your hands and feet?
  —Can you feel me touching your hands and feet?
  —Are you experiencing any tingling and where do you feel this?
- Evaluate for the following:
  —Contusions
  —Deformities
  —Lacerations
  —Punctures
  —Impaled objects
  —Swelling
- Immobilize the patient's head and neck.
- Perform the primary assessment:
  —Airway
  —Breathing
  —Circulation
- Check the patient's vital signs every 2 minutes.
- Control the patient's bleeding.
- Assess the patient's mental status.
- Keep the patient talking.
- Reassure the patient by explaining any required procedures.
- Check for paralysis and weakness in strength by having the patient squeeze your hand or hold an item.
- Transport with the weak extremity well padded for protection. Immobilize the extremity by securing it to the body.

# 5. Assessment—Unconscious Patient

- Get information from bystanders about what happened.
- Evaluate for the following:
  —Contusions
  —Deformities
  —Lacerations
  —Punctures
  —Impaled objects
  —Swelling
- Perform the primary assessment:
  —Airway
  —Breathing
  —Circulation
- Check for pulse in the extremities.
- Check vital signs every 2 minutes.
- Control the patient's bleeding.
- Immobilize extremities with deformities.

**APNEA**

- Perform the primary assessment:
  —Airway
  —Breathing
  —Circulation

# 6. Burns

## SUBJECTIVE/OBJECTIVE

Burns are classified into four categories, depending on the agent or source of the burn.

- Electrical
  —Alternating current, direct current, and lighting
- Thermal
  —Fire, steam, hot liquids, and hot objects
- Radiation
  —Ultraviolet rays and nuclear source
- Chemical
  —Acids, bases, and caustic

## DEPTH OF BURN

- Superficial burn (first-degree burn)
  —Only the epidermis is involved
  —Pain
  —Reddening of skin
  —Swelling
  —Example: sunburn
- Partial-thickness burn (second-degree burn)
  —The epidermis and the dermis are involved
  —Pain
  —Reddening of the skin
  —Blisters
- Full-thickness burn (third-degree burn)
  —All the layers of the skin are damaged
  —Skin is charred black
  —Pain if nerves are not involved/destroyed
  —No pain if associated with nerve damage

—Depth of burn could involve muscles and bones
—Skin grafting is required
—Scars are visible upon healing

## SEVERITY OF BURN

- Source of the burn
  —The degree of burn
- Body regions burned
  —Depth of the burn
  —Extent of the burn

## RULE OF NINES

- The amount of burn to the body is calculated by percentages.
- Rule of Nines is a method of estimating the area burned to determine the amount of burn to the body.
  —Sum of the percentages of burns = Total amount of burn to the body

## ASSESSMENT/PLAN

### Electrical Burns

- Shut down electrical current to the area, especially if a live wire is on top of the patient. Do not touch the patient if electricity is still passing through him or her.
- Perform primary assessment:
  —Airway
  —Breathing
  —Circulation
- Prepare to perform CPR.
- Treat for shock.
- Maintain spinal immobility—spinal injuries.

- Contact of electrical site—Look for Entrance wound.
- Location of electricity leaving body—Look for Exit wound.
- Apply a dry, loose sterile dressing to the entrance and exit sites of burn.

    In an electrical burn, the problem is not the burn but the electricity. Electrical current travels through the body by means of blood vessels and gravity. Therefore, current travels through the heart and CPR is recommended.

## ASSESSMENT/PLAN

### Thermal Burns and Radiation Burns
- Perform primary assessment:
  —Airway
  —Breathing
  —Circulation
- Prepare to perform CPR.
- Remove loose clothing from the person while pouring a steady stream of water over him or her, unless the clothing is stuck to the skin. **Do not remove the clothing from the skin.**
- Treat for shock.
- Treat for dehydration.
- Apply a dry, loose sterile dressing to the burn area.
- Do not break blisters—the possibility of infection increases.

## ASSESSMENT/PLAN

### Chemical Burns
- Perform primary assessment:
  —Airway
  —Breathing
  —Circulation

- Prepare to perform CPR.
- Wash away the chemical with lots of water.
- If the chemical is dry, brush it away as much as possible. Then use a steady flow of water to remove the chemical. Wash for 20 minutes.
- Remove clothing while the water is washing off the chemicals from the body.
- Apply loose sterile dressing.
- Document all findings concerning the patient's condition.

# 7. Cardiac Pain (Chest Pain) with Possible Cardiac Arrest (MI, Myocardial Infarction)/ Congestive Heart Failure

## CAUSES OF CARDIAC COMPROMISE

- Coronary artery disease
  —Atherosclerosis
  —Thrombus
  —Occlusion
  —Embolism
- Aneurysm
- Electrical malfunctions of the heart
  —Dysrhythmia
- Mechanical malfunction of the heart
- Angina pectoris
- Acute myocardial infarction
- Congestive heart failure

## SUBJECTIVE/OBJECTIVE

- Nature of pain
- Onset of pain
- Shortness of breath
- Difficulty in breathing
- Nausea/vomiting
- Diaphoresis (profuse sweating)
- Palpitations
- Anxiety

Cardiac Pain

15

## ASSESSMENT/EVALUATION

- Give oxygen as per the physician's orders.
- Perform an electro cardiogram (EKG) and give results to the physician.
- Perform glucose monitor test to check the level of glucose in the blood.
- Ask if the patient has had any surgeries in the past 6 months:
  —Ask the reason for the surgeries.
- Check vital signs every 2 minutes.

## PLAN

- Inform the physician of the subjective and the objective findings of the patient.
- Obtain a crash cart.
- Maintain oxygen flow as per the physician's order.
- Check vital signs every 2 minutes.
- Give medications as per the physician's order.
- Monitor the level of consciousness and deteriorating conditions.
- Perform primary assessment:
  —Airway
  —Breathing
  —Circulation
- Do not leave the patient alone.
- Document all findings and treatment concerning the patient's condition and evaluation.

# 8. *Chest Wounds*

## TYPES OF CHEST INJURIES

- Blunt trauma
  —Blow to the chest
  —Fractured ribs
  —Damaged lungs and airway
  —Injured heart
- Penetrating objects
  —Bullets
  —Knives
  —Objects that can penetrate the skin
    - Entrance wound and possibly an exit
      wound
- Compression
  —Chest compressed
  —Heart squeezed
  —Lungs ruptured
    - As a result of the chest hitting the steering wheel of
      a car

## SUBJECTIVE/OBJECTIVE

All open wounds to the chest are life threatening.
Penetrating puncture wounds penetrate the chest wall
once. A perforating puncture wound has an entrance and
an exit wound. The object penetrating the skin within the
chest can remain as an impaled object.

When air enters the chest cavity, the pressure within
is greatly decreased. This is why the lungs collapse.

## OPEN CHEST INJURIES

- The chest wall is penetrated
- Object penetrates the skin
- Ribs may be fractured
- Heart, lungs, and vessels are injured
  —Penetrating or perforating puncture wounds

## OPEN CHEST WOUNDS

Occlusive dressing
- One corner of the dressing is left unsealed to the skin—three-sided dressing.
- When the patient inhales, the dressing will seal to the skin.
- When the patient exhales, the unsealed corner will act as a flutter valve releasing the air trapped in the chest cavity.
- This will regulate the respiration.
- If blood accumulates under the dressing, remove the dressing, wipe away the blood, and reseal the dressing on three sides—a flutter-valve dressing.

## CLOSED CHEST INJURIES

- The skin is not perforated.
- Internal bleeding is life threatening.
- Contusions are present.
- Lacerations of the heart, lungs, and vessels may be evident.

## CHEST INJURY COMPLICATIONS

- Pneumothorax
  —Respiratory difficulty
  —Shock

—Distended neck veins
—Uneven chest wall movement
—Reduction of breath sounds
* Hemothorax
  —Same signs and symptoms as pneumothorax, but the patient coughs up blood
* Asphyxia
  —Distended neck veins
  —Skin of head, neck, and shoulders cyanotic
  —Lips cyanotic
* Cardiac tamponade
  —Distended neck veins
  —Weak pulse
  —Low blood pressure
  —Decreasing pulse pressure

## ASSESSMENT/PLAN

* Perform primary assessment:
  —Airway
  —Breathing
  —Circulation
* Prepare to treat for shock.
* Document all findings concerning the patient's condition.

# 9. Diabetic Emergencies

## TYPES OF DIABETES
- Type 1—insulin-dependent diabetes
- Type 2—non–insulin-dependent diabetes
- Hyperglycemia—high blood sugar
- Hypoglycemia—low blood sugar

## SUBJECTIVE/OBJECTIVE
- History of diabetes and current medications
- Increased exercise
- Current symptoms or complaint
- Decreased oral intake
- Last meal
- Last use of insulin
- Status
- Intoxicated appearance
- Cold, clammy skin
- Elevated heart rate
- Uncharacteristic behavior; e.g., combative
- Anxiety
- Seizures

## ASSESSMENT/EVALUATION
- Check vital signs every 2 minutes.
- Evaluate the level of consciousness.
- Check odor of breath.
- Perform glucose monitor test to check the level of glucose in the blood.
- Perform an EKG and give findings to the physician.

## PLAN

- Inform the physician of the subjective and objective findings of the patient.
- Give medications as per the physician's order.
- If hypoglycemic, give sugar-based food or drink to the patient.
- Monitor the level of consciousness.
- Perform primary assessment:
  —Airway
  —Breathing
  —Circulation
- Check vital signs every 2 minutes.
- Document all findings and treatment concerning the glucose levels of the patient.

# 10. Dyspnea/Apnea

## SUBJECTIVE/OBJECTIVE

- Shortness of breath
- Tightness in chest
- Restlessness
- Anxiety
- Increased pulse rate
- Changes in breathing rate
- Changes in breathing rhythm
- Pale, cyanotic, or flushed skin
- Breathing with lung sounds
- High-pitched sounds upon inspiration—upper airway obstruction
- Wheezes—high-pitched sounds, musical in nature
- Crackles—crackling or bubbling sound—fluid in alveoli
- Snoring or rattling sounds
- Stridor
- Rhonchi
- Inability to speak because of breathing difficulty
- Labored breathing/barrel chest
- Level of consciousness
- Coughing
- Flared nostrils
- Patient sitting forward
- Unable to breath in adequate air
- Trauma involved

# 11. Dyspnea (Asthma/ Chronic Obstructive Pulmonary Disease (COPD)/Hypoventilation/ Pulmonary Edema)

## SUBJECTIVE/OBJECTIVE

- Onset of symptoms
  —Slow breathing
  —Rapid respiration
  —Any recent injuries
- Medical history
  —COPD
  —Asthma
  —History of allergic reaction
- Symptoms
  —Chest pain
  —Dyspnea
  —Cough
  —Fever
  —Chills
  —Edema
  —Paresthesia

## ASSESSMENT/EVALUATION

- Evaluate the level of consciousness.
- Check vital signs every 2 minutes.

- Perform an EKG and give evaluation to the physician.
- Perform neurological evaluation:
  —Evidence of drug and/or alcohol intake

## PLAN
- Inform the physician of the subjective and objective findings of the patient.
- Give breathing exercises as per the physician's order.
- Check vital signs after breathing exercise every 2 minutes.
- Watch the patient for any change in respiration because of breathing exercise.
- Perform primary assessment:
  —Airway
  —Breathing
  —Circulation
- Give oxygen as per the physician's order.
- Transport patient in the position of comfort—legs dangling, leaning forward.
- Document all findings and treatment concerning the patient's respiratory evaluation.

# 12. Emergency Medical Phone Calls

As a health care provider, you must be able to differentiate between routine calls and emergencies. Determine the patient's name, location, telephone number, and nature of the emergency. Get this information as quickly as possible because the line may get disconnected or the patient may be unable to continue the conversation.

- Document the following in the patient's chart:
  - —Chief complaint—the emergency stated in the patient's own words
  - —Any known allergies
  - —Illness and injuries the patient has been treated for in the past
  - —Surgical procedures in the past 6 months
  - —What the patient was doing before the illness or the injury occurred?
- Inform the physician of the phone call and communicate the physician's recommendations to the patient.
  - —Is the patient coming into the physician's office or going to the emergency room?
  - —Inform the physician where the patient will receive treatment.
  - —Is there any follow-up?
- You can advise the patient to go to the emergency room immediately.
- You can also call emergency medical service (EMS) to pick up the patient. Stay on the phone with the patient until EMS arrives.

- Remember the following guidelines when dealing with an emergency, whether on the phone or in the office:
  —Stay calm
  —Reassure the patient
  —Act in a confident, organized manner
  —Be professional

# 13. Encephalalgia/ Headache

## SUBJECTIVE/OBJECTIVE
- Onset of symptoms—sudden or gradual
- Current symptoms
- Location of pain
- Nausea/vomiting
- Photophobia
- Fever

## MEDICAL HISTORY
- Subarachnoid hemorrhages
- Any recent trauma to the body
- Migraine headaches
- Exposure to carbon monoxide
- Meningitis
- Medication
- Allergies
- Illicit drug use

## ASSESSMENT/EVALUATION
- Check the patient's vital signs.
- Perform secondary assessment:
  —Neck—stiffness
  —Skin—any rashes
- Evaluate level of consciousness:
  —Deteriorating mental status

## PLAN

- Inform the physician of the subjective and objective findings of the patient.
- Perform primary assessment:
  —Airway
  —Breathing
  —Circulation
- Maintain airway.
- Give medications as per the physician's order.
- Lower the light in the room.
- Keep the patient and family calm.
- Move quietly around the room.
- Place the patient in a position of comfort.
- Document all findings concerning with the condition of the patient.

# 14. External Bleeding

## SUBJECTIVE/OBJECTIVE

### Arteries
* Oxygen-rich blood
* Blood spurts
* Bright red in color

### Veins
* Low-oxygen blood
* Blood runs steady
* Dark red or maroon in color

### Capillaries
* Oxygen-rich blood from the arteries, to supply all cells
* Blood runs slow
* Between bright red and maroon in color

### Pressure Points
* Profuse bleeding of an extremity
  —Upper extremity
    – Brachial artery
  —Lower extremity
    – Femoral artery

Pressure points are used only when direct pressure does not stop the bleeding.

## ASSESSMENT/PLAN

* Direct pressure:
  —Use a dressing and continue to add dressings.
  —Do not remove the other dressings applied.

—Do not waste time; use a gloved hand to apply direct pressure.
- Elevation:
  —Elevate limb above the heart.
- Pressure points:
  —Apply pressure at a pressure point—a large artery that lies close to the surface of the skin and directly over a bone.
- Perform primary assessment:
  —Airway
  —Breathing
  —Circulation
- Document all findings concerning the patient's condition.

# 15. Fever

## SUBJECTIVE/OBJECTIVE
- Onset of additional symptoms
  —Nausea/vomiting
  —Headache
  —Level of consciousness
  —Rash
  —Diarrhea
  —Dehydration
  —Heat disorder—due to weather conditions
- Medical history
  —Has the patient been sick recently?
  —Has the patient undergone any recent surgeries?
  —Has the patient been outside in extreme heat
    conditions?
- Medications
  —Age of the patient

## ASSESSMENT/EVALUATION
- Check core temperature.
- Evaluate the level of consciousness.
- Check turgor of the skin for dehydration.
- Check for signs of seizures.
- Check the patient's vital signs.

## PLAN
- Inform the physician of the subjective and objective
  findings of the patient.
- Loosen the patient's clothing.

- Place cool, wet towels on the patient's forehead.
- Give medications as per the physician's order.
- Check the patient's vital signs.
- Observe the patient's level of consciousness at all times and inform the physician of any changes.
- Provide patient education for any take-home medications or treatment.
- Document all findings and treatment concerning the core temperature and the level of consciousness of the patient.

Fever

# 16. Hypertension

## SUBJECTIVE/OBJECTIVE
- HTN medications
- Medical history
  —Headache
  —Nausea/vomiting
  —Blurred vision
  —Chest pain
  —Dyspnea
- Weakness
  —Tinnitus—ringing in the ears
  —Epistaxis—nosebleed

## ASSESSMENT/EVALUATION
- Check vital signs.
- Evaluate the level of consciousness.
- Determine the degree of chest pain.
- Perform an EKG and give the findings to the physician.

## PLAN
- Inform the physician of the subjective and objective findings of the patient.
- Perform primary assessment:
  —Airway
  —Breathing
  —Circulation
- Give oxygen as per the physician's order.

- Give medication as per the physician's order.
- Check vital signs every 2 minutes.
- Monitor the level of consciousness.
- Document all findings and treatment concerning the patient's hypertension.

# 17. Hyperthermia/Heat Exhaustion/Heat Stroke

## SIGNS AND SYMPTOMS

- Muscle cramps
- Weakness
- Exhaustion
- Rapid, shallow breathing
- Weak pulse
- Heavy perspiration
- Lack of perspiration
- Loss of consciousness

## SUBJECTIVE/OBJECTIVE

- Heat exposure
- Athletic event
- Duration of time in heat
- Clothing worn
- Environment
- Presence or absence of sweat
- Symptoms such as:
  —Nausea/vomiting
- Fluid intake
  —What is the amount of fluid intake?
  —What kinds of fluids did the patient drink?
  —How often were they taken?
- Medical history
  —History of heat stroke
- Medication taken

## ASSESSMENT/EVALUATION

- Check vital signs.
- Give fluids.
- Evaluate the level of consciousness.
- Perform secondary assessment:
  —Evaluate for injuries.
  —Check skin turgor—dehydration.
- Perform glucose monitor test to check glucose level in the blood.
- Perform an EKG and give the findings to the physician.

## PLAN

- Inform the physician of the subjective and objective findings of the patient.
- Maintain airway.
- Give oxygen if patient has dyspnea.
- Check the level of consciousness—deterioration of mental status can cause further damage to the rest of the body (heat stroke).
- Perform primary assessment:
  —Airway
  —Breathing
  —Circulation
- Remove the patient from the heat source and place in an air-conditioned room.
- Remove clothing.
- Place cool towels on the patient's forehead and around the back of the neck.
- Assist the physician with any medications or treatments.
- Allow the patient to assume a position of comfort.
- Check vital signs every 2 minutes.
- Document all findings and treatment concerning the patient's condition.

# 18. Hyperventilation

Hyperventilation is associated with the following:
* Asthma
* Pulmonary embolism
* Edema
* Anxiety attacks
* Allergic reactions
    Document all findings and treatment concerning the patient's evaluation.

## ASSESSMENT/EVALUATION
* Perform an EKG and give findings to the physician.
* Evaluate the level of consciousness.
* Ask about trauma/medical history.
* Ask if the patient has a history of COPD.
* Ask if the patient has any allergies.
* Ask when did the patient ate.
* Ask what was eaten. Choking may be present.
* Let the patient sit in a position of comfort, with legs dangling, leaning forward.

## PLAN
* Inform the physician of subjective and objective findings of the patient.
* Perform primary assessment:
    —Airway
    —Breathing
    —Circulation
* Monitor for choking.

- Give oxygen as per the physician's order.
- Check vital signs every 2 minutes.
- Assist the patient in taking medications as per the physician's order.
- Transport the patient in a position of comfort, with legs dangling, leaning forward.
- Automated external defibrillator (AED).

Stop CPR and apply the pads of the AED. The monitor will guide you through the process of administering shock or continuing with CPR.

- Document all findings and treatment concerning the patient's respiratory condition.

# 19. Hypothermia/ Frostbite

## SIGNS AND SYMPTOMS

- Shivering
- Difficulty speaking
- Muscular rigidity
- Irrational
- Unconscious

## SUBJECTIVE/OBJECTIVE

- Clothing worn
- Environment
- Length of exposure
- Symptoms such as:
  —Pain
  —Numbness
  —Shivering (muscle cramps)
  —Altered level of consciousness
  —Mental status
    – Is the patient able to identify surroundings?
    – Is the patient able to answer simple questions?
- Medication taken

## ASSESSMENT/EVALUATION

- Perform primary assessment:
  —Airway
  —Breathing
  —Circulation

- Check vital signs.
- Check core temperature of the body (hypothermia = core temperature less than 95°F).
- Evaluate the level of consciousness.
- Perform an EKG and give findings to the physician.
- Evaluate extremities for the presence or absence of sweat:
  —Temperature
  —Capillary refill—due to circulation
  —Sensation—Can the patient feel pressure in the extremities?
  —Frostbite
  —Secondary assessment—Are there any further injuries?

## PLAN

- Inform the physician of the subjective and objective findings of the patient.
- Passive rewarming:
  —When the body rewarms itself?
- Active rewarming:
  —Application of an external heat source to the body
- Check vital signs every 2 minutes.
- Perform primary assessment:
  —Airway
  —Breathing
  —Circulation
- Evaluate the level of consciousness—deterioration of the mental status can cause further damage to the body.
- Avoid rough handling of the patient, because he or she is subject to cardiac arrhythmias.
- Remove any wet clothing.
- Place warm packs in the patient's axilla and groin area.
- Give warm fluids—by mouth (PO).

- Bundle the patient in warm blankets or sleeping bag.
- Frostbitten extremities in clean sterile dressing.
- Transport to a facility with invasive rewarming capabilities (intravenous four (IV) therapy—done only by physician or someone with IV therapy certification).
- Document all findings and treatment concerning the hypothermia of the patient.

# 20. Injuries to the Skull, Brain, and Facial Bones

- The scalp has many blood vessels, which will bleed profusely when injured.
- If injury to the scalp is severe, there could be fractures of the cranium and/or the facial bones.
- Fractures could be severe enough to damage the brain and may interfere with the airway for breathing.
- There may be open or closed wounds.

## BRAIN INJURIES

- Direct injuries
- Open head injuries
- Brain with lacerations, punctures, or contusions because of broken bones or foreign objects
- Indirect injuries
- Open or closed wounds
- Shock of impact on the skull transferred to the brain
- Shaken baby syndrome (infants and children get so traumatized by the physical shaking that the brain tissue within the skull tends to move around within the cranium)
- Concussions
- Contusions

## Types of Brain Injuries
- Concussion

—A fall or a hit by an object (the force is transferred
  through the skull to the brain)
—Headache
—Conscious
—Unconscious
—Possible loss of memory
—Dazed
—Pain at the site of impact
- Contusion
  —The force of the blow is great enough to rupture the
    blood vessels within the brain
  —Closed/open head injuries
    – Internal and/or external bleeding
  —The blow to the head causes the brain to hit the inside
    of the skull
- Laceration or puncture wound
  —An object penetrating the cranium may cause a
    puncture wound
  —The bones of the skull could cut the brain
    – Hit with an object
    – Puncture wound
- Hematoma
  —Collection of blood within the tissue
    – Subdural hematoma—collection of blood between
      the brain and the dura of the brain
    – Epidural hematoma—blood between the dura and
      the skull
    – Intracerebral hematoma—when the blood
      surrounds the brain

**Subjective/Objective**
- Visible bone fragments
- Altered mental status
- Lacerations
- Hematoma

- Deformity of the skull
- Pain
- Hematoma behind the ear
- Pupils equal and unreactive to light
- Discoloration around the eyes (black eyes)
- Cerebrospinal fluid from the ears
- Bleeding from the nose or ears
- Personality change; e.g., irritable
- Increased blood pressure
- Decreased pulse rate
- Irregular breathing patterns
- Blurred vision in both eyes

## IMPALED OBJECTS IN CRANIUM

- Do not remove the impaled object.
- Stabilize the object.
- Pad around the object with bulky dressings.

## INJURIES TO THE FACE

- Immobilize the head and neck.
- Perform primary assessment:
  —Airway
  —Breathing
  —Circulation
- Maintain the patency of the airway because of likely obstruction from bone fragments.
- Perform jaw-thrust maneuver to open airway to begin CPR.
- Clear blood from the throat as that can be an obstruction.
- Soak teeth that have fallen out in milk and transport with the patient.

- Fracture in the mandible
  —Patient is unable to move the lower jaw.
  —Improper alignment of the upper and lower jaw.
  —Bleeding around the teeth.
  —Perform jaw-thrust maneuver to open airway
  for CPR.

## INJURIES TO THE SPINE

Spinal injuries can be related to other injuries of the body.
These are associated with head, neck, and back injury. If
a cervical collar is available, position it appropriately. If a
cervical collar is not available, immobilize the patient from
head to toe in one straight-line supine position. Use all
bystanders available for help.

    Most spinal injuries are due to:
- Compression injuries
- Excessive flexion, extension and rotation from falls
- Diving injuries
- Motor vehicle accidents
- Sports accidents—player contact and falling to the
  ground
- Any fall from three times the patient's height can cause:
  —Open fractures of the ankle
  —Spinal damage
- Skating injuries
- Mountain biking injuries
- Surfing injuries
- Mountain climbing and rock climbing accidents
- Sledding and skiing accidents

### Subjective/Objective
- Paralysis of the extremities
- Pain without movement
- Pain with movement

- Tenderness in the spine
- Impaired breathing
- Postural deformity
- Weakness, tingling, or loss of sensation in the upper or lower extremities
- Spinal shock—neurological
- Soft tissue injuries

**Assessment/Plan**
- If a cervical collar is available, use proper placement.
- Immobilize the head and neck.
- Perform primary assessment:
  —Airway
  —Breathing
  —Circulation
- Check vital signs every 2 minutes.
- Control bleeding: apply direct pressure and a loose sterile bandage.
- Bandage all wounds.
- Talk to conscious patient.
- Treat for shock.
- Document all findings concerning the patient's condition.

# 21. Internal Bleeding

- Damage to the internal organs or vessels
- Blood loss that cannot be seen
- Injury to the extremities

## SUBJECTIVE/OBJECTIVE

- Injury to the surface of the body
- Bruising
- Swelling or deformity of extremity
- Bleeding from the mouth, nose, ear, or other orifices
- Signs and symptoms of shock—hypovolemic

## ASSESSMENT/PLAN

- Control external bleeding.
- Prepare to treat for shock.
- Do not let the patient lean back—he or she will choke on the blood.
- If patient is unconscious—place in recovery position.
- Perform primary assessment:
  —Airway
  —Breathing
  —Circulation
- Maintain airway.
- Check vital signs every 2 minutes.
- Document all findings concerning the patient's condition.

# 22. Musculoskeletal Injuries

## TYPES OF MUSCULOSKELETAL INJURIES

- Fractures
  —Any break in the bone
- Dislocations
  —The joint coming out of the socket
- Sprains
  —Stretching or tearing of the ligament
- Strains
  —Overexertion or overstretching of the muscle
- Closed extremity injury (simple)
  —Injury to extremity with no exposure
- Open extremity injury (compound)
  —Injury to extremity with the skin exposing the injury

## SUBJECTIVE/OBJECTIVE

- Pain
- Deformity
- Sound of bones rubbing together
- Swelling
- Bruising
- Exposed bones
- Bleeding

## ASSESSMENT/PLAN

- Primary assessment pertaining to internal bleeding.
- Femur injuries can be fatal because of internal bleeding.

- In trauma cases—immobilize head and neck (apply cervical collar).
- Secure the injured part and immobilize using splint.
- Check for pulse; if no pulse, loosen splint.
- Place cold pack on the site of injury to reduce swelling.
- Apply a loose sterile dressing to cover open musculoskeletal injury.

## DISLOCATIONS

- Shoulder dislocation—Sling the arm of the dislocation upward on the chest. Then secure the arm and hand to the body. This will reduce the pain. Make sure there is a radial pulse. If there is no pulse, loosen sling.
- Hip dislocation—Immobilize hip with pillows and rolled blankets. Check for pedal pulse. Due to possible internal bleeding, treat for shock.
- Perform primary assessment:
  —Airway
  —Breathing
  —Circulation
- Document all findings concerning the patient's condition.

# 23. Nausea/Vomiting

## SUBJECTIVE/OBJECTIVE

- Onset of symptoms
- Frequency
- Duration
- Contents of emesis
- Any blood
- Symptoms of fever, chills, pain, and weakness
- Medical history
- Medications
- Illness
- Surgery

## ASSESSMENT/EVALUATION

- Maintain airway.
- Check vital signs.
- Assess the level of consciousness.
- Assess for signs of dehydration—check skin turgor.
- Perform glucose monitor test to check blood glucose level.
- Check for blood in emesis.
- Secondary assessment—abdominal evaluation:
  —Pain
  —Guarding
  —Distention

## PLAN

- Inform the physician of the subjective and objective findings of the patient.

- Treat for shock.
- Check vital signs.
- Check the level of consciousness.
- Assist the patient with taking medications.
- Possible IV therapy done only by physician or someone with IV therapy certification, for dehydration.
- Give patient education for medication and treatment.
- Document all findings concerning the patient's condition.

# 24. Poisoning and Overdose—Toxic Ingestion

## ROUTE OF ENTRY

Poisons can be:
- Ingested
- Inhaled
- Absorbed
- Injected

## COMMON POISONS

- Cough and cold medications
- Aspirin
- Food poisoning
- Insecticides
- Petroleum products
- Acetaminophen
- Acids and alkalis
- Antihistamines
- Plants

### Questions to Ask the Patient
- What substance is involved?
- When did the exposure occur?
- How much was ingested?
- What antidotes were given, if any?
- What is the weight of the patient?
- What are the effects that the patient is experiencing?

- Call Poison Control Center.
- Call 911 and give information.


## SUBJECTIVE/OBJECTIVE

- History of ingestion:
  —What?
  —When?
  —How much?
- Symptoms such as:
  —Burning sensations
  —Nausea/vomiting
  —Sleepiness
- Type and duration of exposure
- Medical history and medications
- Medications or drugs the patient could have taken
- Actions before ingestion
- Was vomiting induced?
- Other medications or food given?
- Patient's history:
  —Suicidal intent ingestion
  —Other harmful action to self
  —Medical and psychiatric history

## ASSESSMENT/EVALUATION

- Maintain airway.
- Perform an EKG and give findings to the physician.
- Check for medical alert tags.
- Be alert for signs of intoxication or drug use.
- Check the odor of the patient's breath.
- Assess the patient's level of consciousness and neurologic responses.
- Check vital signs every 2 minutes.

- Respiratory examination: How is the patient breathing?
- Prepare to start CPR.
- Call 911.

**PLAN**
- Inform the physician of the objective and subjective findings of the patient.
- Perform primary assessment:
  —Airway
  —Breathing
  —Circulation
- Do not induce vomiting unless specified by the physician or Poison Control Center. If the patient ingested a petroleum product, vomiting will do more damage to the patient.
- Assist the physician with medication and treatment.
- Consider involving the police if the patient becomes hostile.
- Be cautious of weapons.
- Inform EMS and police of any change in behavior or anything unusual.
- Attempt to establish a rapport with the patient. Do not get yourself hurt in the meantime.
- Be professional and courteous.
- Document all findings and treatment concerning the patient's condition.

# 25. Pulmonary Embolism Suspected

## SUBJECTIVE/OBJECTIVE

- Symptoms:
  —Chest pain
  —Dyspnea
  —Leg swelling
  —Pain
- Medical history:
  —Prior pulmonary embolism
  —Known clotting disorder
  —Prior deep vein thrombosis
  —Any recent surgery
- Medications
  —Blood-thinning medications such as Coumadin are being taken by the patient.
  —Patient is no longer taking the blood-thinning medications.
  —Is there any known history of allergy?

## ASSESSMENT/EVALUATION

- Maintain airway patency.
- Check vital signs.
- Assess the level of consciousness.
- Perform an EKG and give findings to the physician.

## PLAN

- Inform the physician of the subjective and objective findings of the patient.
- Perform primary assessment:
  —Airway
  —Breathing
  —Circulation
- Give oxygen as per the physician's order.
- Check vital signs every 2 minutes.
- Transport patient in the position of comfort—usually at a 45° angle sitting position.

# 26. Respirations

**Rate**
- Adult 12–20/minute
- Child 15–30/minute
- Infant 25–50/minute

**Rhythm**
- Regular

**Quality**
- Breath sounds
  —Present and equal
- Chest expansion
  —Adequate and equal
- Effort of breathing
- Unlabored, normal respiratory effort
- Depth
  —Adequate

## QUESTIONS TO ASK THE PATIENT

### OPQRST
- Onset—When did it begin?
- Provocation—What was the patient doing when this started?
- Quality—Describe the feeling.
- Radiation—Does the pain radiate to other parts of the body?
- Severity—On a scale of 1–10, with 10 being the worst—How bad are the pains?
- Time—How long has this feeling been present?

# 27. Seizure

## CONVULSIVE SEIZURES

Convulsive seizures are associated with the following:
- Epilepsy
- Stroke
- Measles, mumps, and other childhood diseases
- Hypoglycemia
- Eclampsia—pregnancy
- Hypoxia
- Heat stroke
Seizures in children
- Toxic—drug or alcohol abuse
- Brain tumor
- Congenital birth defects
- Fever—infection
- Metabolic
- Trauma

## TYPES OF SEIZURES

- Grand mal—tonic clonic
  —Breathing may stop
  —Body becomes stiff
  —Biting of the tongue
  —Uncontrollable bowel
- Clonic phase
  —Jerks about violently
  —Foaming of the mouth
  —Drooling
  —Cyanotic skin

58

- Postictal Phase
    —Cessation of convulsion
    —Consciousness
    —Drowsiness
    —Confusion
- Simple partial seizure
    —Tingling, stiffening, and jerking of one part of the body
    —Aura—smell, bright lights, colors
    —No loss of consciousness
- Complex partial seizure
    —Aura
    —Abnormal behavior
    —Confusion
    —Glassy stare
    —Person appears to be drunk or on drugs
    —No memory of the episode

Health care providers cannot diagnose the type of seizure the patient is experiencing. They can use this information to give the physician more information in their report on the patient.

## SUBJECTIVE/OBJECTIVE

History of seizures
- Onset
- Duration
- Type of seizure—grand mal/petit mal
- Trauma before seizure or related to seizure
- Fever

## MEDICAL HISTORY

- Previous seizure disorder
- Current medications

- History of "breakthrough" seizures
- Drug or alcohol use
- Pregnancy

## ASSESSMENT/EVALUATION

Check the following:
- Vital signs
- Level of consciousness
- Any oral trauma
- Trauma in the neck
- Evidence of incontinence
- Evidence of alcohol or drug use
- Secondary survey—looking for injuries

## PLAN

- Inform the physician of the objective and subjective findings of the patient concerning seizures and the level of consciousness of the patient.
- Perform primary assessment:
  —Airway
  —Breathing
  —Circulation
- Do not use a bite stick or attempt to put anything in the mouth.
- Protect the patient's head from any trauma during a seizure.
- Keep all objects away from the patient.
- Do not restrain the patient during a seizure.
- Place the patient on the left side—recovery position.

- Spinal injury—immobilize the patient:
  —Supine position
  —Cervical collar applied
- Inform EMS of all findings.
- Document all information concerning the seizure
  and any other injuries.

# 28. Shock

## THREE CATEGORIES OF SHOCK

- Compensated shock
  —The body attempts to compensate for the loss
    of blood in the vessels.
  —Early signs of shock.
  —Blood pressure maintained.
  —Increased heart rate.
  —Increased respirations.
- Decompensated shock
  —The body can no longer compensate for the loss
    of blood.
  —Late signs of shock.
  —Falling blood pressure.
- Irreversible shock
  —The body can no longer fight to maintain perfusion to
    the organs. The liver and kidneys begin to shut down.
  —Falling blood pressure, decrease in the vital signs.
  —Washout stage—death due to failure of irreparably
    damaged organs.

## SIGNS AND SYMPTOMS

- Altered mental status.
- Pale, cool, clammy skin.
- Nausea/vomiting.
- Change in vital signs:
  —Pulse increases
  —Respirations increase
  —Blood pressure drops
- Swelling

- Itching
- Thirst
- Weakness
- Edema
- Respiratory distress
- Chest pain
- Dizziness
- Syncope
- Abdominal pain
- Medical history:
  —Drug ingestion
  —Known allergies
  —Diarrhea
  —Recent trauma
  —Last menstrual period
  —Fever
  —Vaginal bleeding
  —Medical surgeries
  —Illnesses
  —Infection

## SUBJECTIVE/OBJECTIVE

- Conscious vs. unconsciousness
- Neck—jugular venous distention
- Pulmonary—wheezes, respiratory effort
- Capillary refill
- Diaphoresis
- Core temperature of the body
- Onset of symptoms:
  —Rapid
  —Gradual
- Known precipitating events

## ASSESSMENT/EVALUATION

- Maintain airway.
- Control external bleeding.
- Place patient in shock position—lift legs above heart, and cover with blanket.
- Check vital signs.
- Assess the level of consciousness.
- Secondary assessment—check for any signs of trauma.

## PLAN

- Inform the physician of the subjective and objective findings of the patient.
- Perform primary assessment:
  —Airway
  —Breathing
  —Circulation
- Give medications as per the physician's orders.
- Place patient in the shock position, with legs elevated slightly above heart.
- Cover with a blanket.
- Do not give the patient food or beverage.
- Check vital signs every 2 minutes.
- Document all findings and treatment concerning the patient.

shock

# 29. *Soft Tissue Injuries*

## SUBJECTIVE/OBJECTIVE

* Closed wounds
  —Contusion—bruise
  —Hematoma—blood under the skin at the injury site
  —Crush injury—internal organs crushed or ruptured and internal bleeding
* Open Wounds
  —Abrasions—scrapes and scratches
  —Lacerations—cuts, smooth or jagged
  —Punctures—sharp, pointed object passes through the skin
  —Avulsions—flaps of skin or tissue torn loose or pulled off completely
  —Amputations—fingers, toes, arms, or legs torn off
  —Crush injuries—internal organs crushed, with external bleeding

## ASSESSMENT/PLAN

* Expose the wound.
* Clean wound—rid any debris from wound/sterile procedure.
* Direct pressure—control bleeding.
* Puncture wound—look for an entrance and an exit wound. Control bleeding from both sites.
* Impaled object—immobilize the object from moving. Do not remove an impaled object if the object is in the facial area, maintain airway at all times.
* Place patient in shock position unless head trauma involved.

- Reassure the patient.
- Perform primary assessment:
  —Airway
  —Breathing
  —Circulation
- Document all findings concerning the patient's condition.

# 30. Syncope/Fainting/Dizziness

## CAUSES OF SYNCOPE

- Hypovolemic causes
  —Low fluid/blood volume
- Metabolic causes
  —Disruption in the brain or surrounding tissue
  —Inner or middle ear infection
- Environmental/toxicological causes
  —Alcohol or drug intoxication
- Cardiovascular causes
  —Tachycardia
  —Low blood pressure
  —High blood pressure

## SUBJECTIVE/OBJECTIVE

- History of event:
  —Onset
  —Duration
  —Activity
  —Precipitating factors
  —Food intake
  —Seizure activity with syncope
  —Conscious vs. unconscious

## SYMPTOMS

- Nausea/vomiting
- Dizziness

- Chest or back pain
- Headache

## ASSESSMENT/EVALUATION

- Check vital signs.
- Perform an EKG and give findings to the physician.
- Perform blood glucose monitor to—check blood glucose level.
- Assess the level of consciousness.
- Secondary assessment—check for signs of trauma.

## PLAN

- Inform the physician of the subjective and objective findings of the patient.
- Perform primary assessment:
  —Airway
  —Breathing
  —Circulation
- Give oxygen as per the physician's order.
- Give medications as per the physician's order.
- Prepare to treat for shock:
  —Maintain airway.
  —Place patient in shock position, with legs elevated slightly above heart.
  —Cover with a blanket.
- Give patient education for medication and treatment if the patient is sent home.
- Document all findings concerning the condition of the patient.

# 31. Transient Ischemic Attack (TIA)/Cerebrovascular Accident (CVA)

## SUBJECTIVE/OBJECTIVE

- Confusion
- Dizziness
- Headache
- Numbness
- Impaired vision
- Elevated BP
- Nausea/vomiting
- Unconsciousness
- Onset, duration, and progression of symptoms
- Associated symptoms such as seizures, trauma
- Medications and allergies
- Medical history

A conscious patient can maintain airway. An unconscious patient cannot maintain airway. Reassess airway and breathing continually. Check vital signs every 2 minutes.

## ASSESSMENT/ EVALUATION

- Is the patient conscious or unconscious?
- Perform an EKG and give findings to the physician.
- Check vital signs every 2 minutes.
- Keep affected limbs of the body from dangling off of the bed or examination table—limbs affected by paralysis will not have any control.

- Ask the patient to smile.
- Ask the patient to close his or her eyes.
- Give the patient something to say—check slurring.
- Ask the patient to move his or her arms.
- Assess the level of consciousness.
- Assess neurological status and report findings to the physician.
- Check for signs of trauma due to falling.
- Check blood glucose level.

## PLAN

- Perform primary assessment:
  —Airway
  —Breathing
  —Circulation
- Inform the physician of the subjective and objective findings of the patient.
- Give oxygen as per the physician's order.
- Give medication as per the physician's order.
- Check vital signs every 2 minutes.
- Assess the level of consciousness.
- Transport patient laying on his or her side, with the affected side down.
- Document the findings and treatment concerning to the disability and the evaluation of the patient.

# 32. Trauma

## SUBJECTIVE/OBJECTIVE

- Cause of events
- Scene safety
- Number of patients
- Prioritize according to injury
- Penetrating trauma:
  —Weapons used
- Secondary to exposure:
  —Type of exposure
  —Chemicals
- Patient complaints
- Position of patient, movement since injury and the level of consciousness
- Other medical conditions of patient
- Drug or alcohol use
- Consider activating regional mass disaster plan—police, fire, and EMS

## ASSESSMENT/EVALUATION

- Assess the level of consciousness.
- Immobilize head and neck.
- Immobilize back and spine.

## PLAN

Treat according to priority of injuries.
- Inform the physician of the subjective and objective findings concerning the trauma of the patient.

- Perform primary assessment:
  —Airway
  —Breathing
  —Circulation
- Check vital signs every 2 minutes.
- Monitor the level of consciousness.
- Assess head, neck, and spinal injuries.
- Assess abdominal injuries.
- Control bleeding.
- Assess nonthreatening injuries.

Prioritize from the most critical or life threatening to the less severe patient.

# INDEX

Index

Index

Index

Index